THE ✚DANIELPLAN FIVE ESSENTIALS SERIES

FITNESS

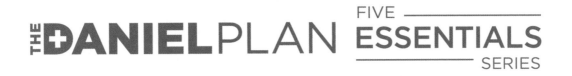

THE DANIEL PLAN FIVE ESSENTIALS SERIES

FITNESS

═══ *Essential Three* ═══

STRENGTHENING YOUR BODY

STUDY GUIDE   FOUR SESSIONS

featuring

SEAN FOY,
BASHEERAH AHMAD,
& DEE EASTMAN
with KAREN LEE-THORP

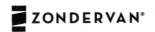

ZONDERVAN

Fitness Study Guide
Copyright © 2015 by The Daniel Plan

This title is also available as a Zondervan ebook. Visit www.zondervan.com/ebooks.

Requests for information should be addressed to:
Zondervan, 3900 *Sparks Dr. SE, Grand Rapids, Michigan 49546*

ISBN 978-0-310-82298-1

Cover photography: iStockphoto
Interior photography: Robert Ortiz, Kent Cameron, Don Haynes, Robert Hawkins, Shelly Antol, Matt Armendariz,
*   the PICS Ministry at Saddleback Church, iStockphoto*
Interior design: Kait Lamphere

First Printing May 2015 / Printed in the United States of America

Contents

Welcome Letter

I am so glad you have joined us for this Daniel Plan study. I am excited for your journey, as I have seen firsthand that change is within reach as you embrace the Daniel Plan lifestyle. This groundbreaking program will equip you with practical tools to bring health into every area of your life. It has been transformative for thousands of people around the world and can be for you as well.

I speak from experience. I've not only witnessed endless stories of life change but have personally benefited from these Daniel Plan Essentials for many years now. Working full-time with five grown children, including identical triplet girls, I understand what it is like to juggle many priorities and have my health impacted. The key elements of The Daniel Plan have been completely restorative in my life as I have integrated them one step at a time.

As you go through this four-week study, the perfect complement to maximize your success is reading *The Daniel Plan: 40 Days to a Healthier Life*. The book includes a 40-day food and fitness guide, complete with a meal plan, recipes, shopping lists, and exercises that will energize your efforts. It will complement any of The Daniel Plan studies you dive into. There are also numerous articles and free resources on our website (www.danielplan.com), along with a weekly newsletter filled with tools and inspiration to keep you flourishing.

Congratulations on taking the next step to gaining vitality in your life. My prayer is that you will be inspired and fully equipped to continue your journey, and that you will experience a whole new level of wellness in the process. I pray that you will feel God's presence and will be reenergized to follow all he has planned for you.

For His Glory,

Dee Eastman

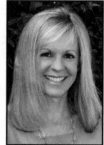

Dee Eastman
Founding Director, The Daniel Plan

How to Use This Guide

There are five video studies in The Daniel Plan series, one for each of the five Essentials (Faith, Food, Fitness, Focus, and Friends). Each study is four sessions long. The studies may be done in any order. If your group is new, consider starting with the six-week *The Daniel Plan Study Guide* and companion DVD, which offers an overview of all five Essentials.

GROUP SIZE

Each Daniel Plan video study is designed to be experienced in a group setting such as a Bible study, Sunday school class, or any small group gathering. To ensure that everyone has enough time to participate in discussions, it is recommended that large groups break into smaller groups of four to six people each.

MATERIALS NEEDED

Each participant should have his or her own study guide, which includes notes for video segments, directions for activities, discussion questions, and ideas for personal application between sessions. This curriculum is best used in conjunction with *The Daniel Plan: 40 Days to a Healthier Life*, which includes a complete 40-day food and fitness guide that complements this study.

TIMING

Each session is designed to be completed in 60 to 90 minutes, depending on your setting and the size of your group. Each video is approximately 20 minutes long.

OUTLINE OF EACH SESSION

Each group session will include the following:

» *Coming Together.* The foundation for spiritual growth is an intimate connection with God and his family. A few people who really know you and earn your trust provide a place to experience the life Jesus invites you to live. This opening portion of your meeting is an opportunity to transition from your busy life into your group time.

   In Session 1 you'll find some icebreaker questions on the session topic, along with guidelines that state the values your group will live by so that everyone feels comfortable sharing. In Sessions 2 – 4 you'll have a chance to check in with other group members to report praise and progress toward your goals of healthy living. You'll also be able to share how you chose to put the previous session's insights into practice – and what the results were. There's no pressure for everyone to answer. This is time to get to know each other better and cheer each other on.

» *Learning Together.* This is the time when you will view the video teaching segment. This study guide provides notes on the key points of the video teaching along with space for you to write additional thoughts and questions.

» *Growing Together.* Here is where you will discuss the teaching you watched. The focus will be on how the teaching intersects with your real life.

» *What I Want to Remember.* You'll have a couple of minutes after your discussion to write down one or two key insights from the teaching and discussion that you want to remember.

» *Better Together.* The Daniel Plan is all about transforming the way you actually live. So before you close your meeting in prayer, you'll take some time to think about how you might apply what you've discussed. Under "Next Steps" you'll find a list of things you can do to put the session's insights into practice. Then the "Food Tip of the Week" offers a bonus video with a great recipe or food idea. It is on your DVD if you want to view it together with your group. It is also available online for you to view on your own during the week. Likewise, the "Fitness Move of the Week" is a bonus video with a simple exercise you can add to your fitness practices. It, too, is on your DVD and online.

Encourage each other to be specific about one or two things you plan to do each week as next steps. Consider asking someone in the group to be your buddy to hold each other accountable. Create an atmosphere of fun and positive reinforcement.

» *Praying Together.* The group session will close with time for a response to God in prayer, thanking him for what he's doing for you and asking for his help to live out what you have learned. Ideas for group prayer, as well as a written closing prayer, are provided. Feel free to use them or not. Consider having different group members lead the prayer time.

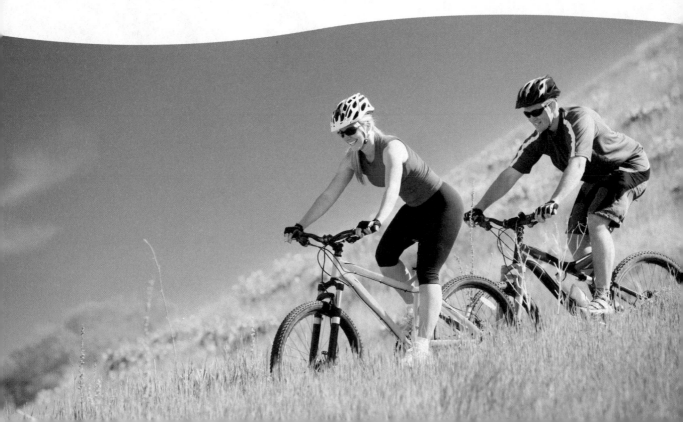

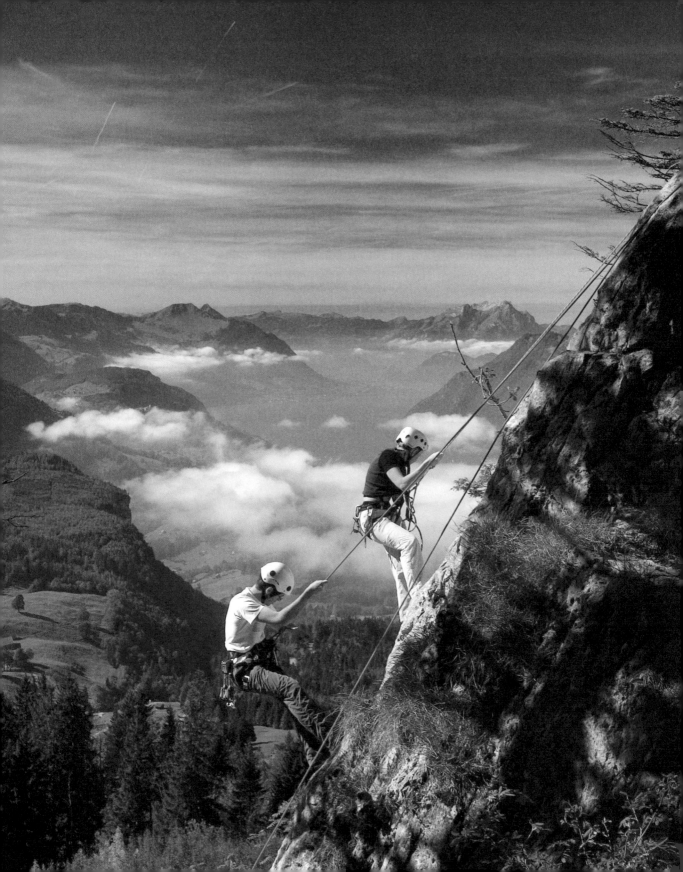

Becoming Daniel Strong

> "Each time [God] said, 'My grace is all you need. My power works best in weakness.' So now I am glad to boast about my weaknesses, so that the power of Christ can work through me."
> 2 Corinthians 12:9 (NLT)

When we think of physical fitness, we may get a picture of a body builder proud of his perfect physique, congratulating himself on his hard work, flexing his muscles as an emblem of his self-sufficiency. That's not what it means to be Daniel Strong, however. Forget the perfection, lose the pride, and dump the self-sufficiency. In this study on Fitness, we'll learn a very different model of strength. We'll begin in this session by looking at Daniel himself, the man in the Bible. What was the source of his strength?

COMING
TOGETHER

If this is your first time meeting together as a group, take a moment to introduce yourself.

Also, pass around a sheet of paper on which each person can write his or her name, address, phone number, and email address. Ask for a volunteer to type up the list and email it to everyone else this week.

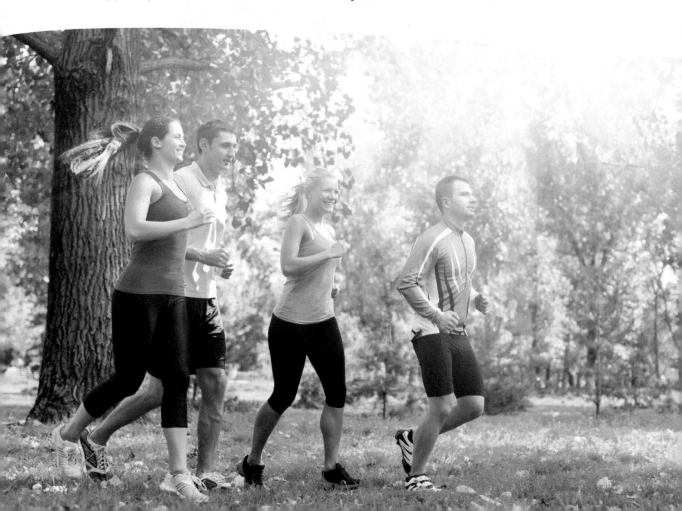

Finally, you'll need some simple group guidelines that outline values and expectations. See the sample in the Appendix and make sure that everyone agrees with and understands those expectations.

When you're finished with these introductory activities, give everyone a chance to answer this icebreaker question:

» What did you enjoy doing physically when you were ten years old? What did "play" look like for you? (Organized team sports, pick-up games, jump rope, freeze tag, riding your bike, make-believe games?) Were there places outside where you liked to play, such as the woods, the sidewalks, or the park?

LEARNING
TOGETHER

Play the video segment for Session 1. As you watch, use the outline provided to follow along or to take additional notes on anything that stands out to you.

» Becoming Daniel Strong means pursuing excellence in body, mind, heart, and soul—all for the glory of God.

» The key to becoming Daniel Strong is the ability to lean on God. Daniel did that. He relied on God's power, not willpower. Self-sufficiency is not desirable.

» Daniel was intentional about his faith, praying three times a day. We can pray in the morning, check in with God at noon to see if we've been relying on God, and check in again at the end of the day.

» Daniel showed his strength by continuing to rely on God through prayer. He showed his strength through a declaration of his weakness and need for God.

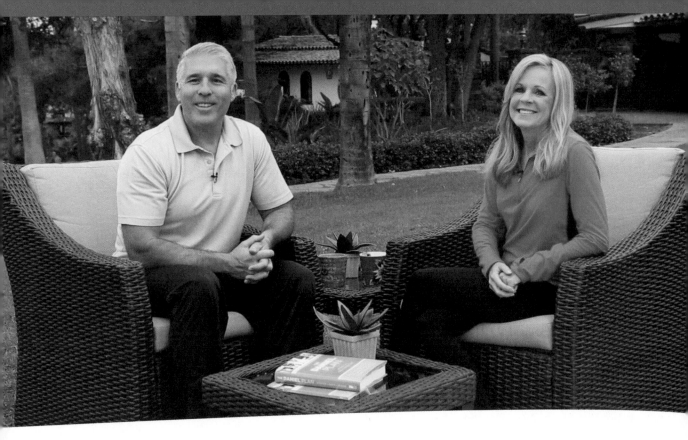

» We can set an alarm to remind us to ask ourselves, "Are you relying on yourself? Or are you relying on God?"

» There's a greater reason to be healthy than just looking good. The greater reason is to be fit to serve God.

» Small steps equal big results. Progress, not perfection.

» We need to cultivate a picture of ourselves as healthy. What would we do for God with our lives if we had the strength?

» The best exercise that will get you in shape is the one you will do. What do you enjoy?

» Identify your fitness personality. Are you a solo exerciser, a social exerciser, or a little of both?

» Schedule your exercise each day like any other appointment.

» Get a buddy to encourage you in your fitness goals.

GROWING
TOGETHER

Discuss what you learned from the video. Don't feel obliged to answer every question. Select those that most resonate with your group.

1 Read Daniel 6:6–10 below. How was Daniel's commitment to prayer—issued after a decree forbidding prayer to anyone but the king—a demonstration of strength? How was it a demonstration of weakness?

"So the administrators and high officers went to the king and said, 'Long live King Darius! We are all in agreement—we administrators, officials, high officers, advisers, and governors—that the king should make a law that will be strictly enforced. Give orders that for the next thirty days any person who prays to anyone, divine or human—except to you, Your Majesty—will be thrown into the den of lions. And now, Your Majesty, issue and sign this law so it cannot be changed, an official law of the Medes and Persians that cannot be revoked.' So King Darius signed the law.

"But when Daniel learned that the law had been signed, he went home and knelt down as usual in his upstairs room, with its windows open toward Jerusalem. He prayed three times a day, just as he had always done, giving thanks to his God."

Daniel 6:6–10 (NLT)

2 Why is it important for us to rely on God for everything, including physical fitness?

3 Take a couple of minutes on your own to ask yourself, "What is my big dream? What would I do to honor God if I were physically fit?" Ask God to guide your thoughts on this. Picture yourself as healthy and fit as you could possibly be. Write your big dream in the space provided, and then share it with the group if you feel comfortable doing so. (If you need a jumpstart, see the box below.)

To inspire you to dream big, here are a few dreams from others who have embarked on The Daniel Plan:

> » Get my blood sugar under control.
> » Feel enthusiastic and energetic when I get out of bed in the morning.
> » Lift my mood and manage my stress.
> » Complete a 5K run.
> » Get a black belt in karate.
> » Learn to swim.
> » Spend an active day with my grandkids without getting exhausted.

> » Cycle across the state with grandkids.
> » Have the energy to actively invest in my marriage.
> » Be healthy enough to get actively involved in ministry.
> » Help build a school in India.
> » Volunteer to coach a kids' softball team.
> » Go on a missions trip with my church.

It's possible that it will take you more than a couple of minutes to identify your big dream. That's okay. It can be a matter for prayer during the coming week. If you don't have an answer for question 3 right now, you can share with the group some of the things you're thinking about. A small dream is a step in the right direction. Do you have a small dream? What goes through your mind when you consider this question of a dream, when you try to picture yourself fit and healthy? Is it hard for you to picture yourself fit enough to do something significant for God? Does the question make you feel hopeful or unhopeful? Why?

What movement do you enjoy? Walking? Swimming? Basketball? Dancing? Mountain climbing? Skateboarding? Racquetball? Trampoline jumping? Skipping rope? If you can't think of something you currently enjoy, what activity could you explore?

6 What goes through your mind when you think about scheduling regular exercise throughout the week? What would help you overcome the barriers to doing that? (For example, could you schedule movement for two or five or ten minutes here and there during the day?)

7 Revisit the subject of relying on God. For what issue related to fitness do you most need to rely on God?

What I Want
to Remember

Complete this activity on your own.

» Briefly review the video outline and any notes you took. Review also any notes from the discussion.

» In the space below, write down the most significant thing you gained from this session—from the video or the discussion. You can share it with the group if you wish.

BETTER
TOGETHER

Now that you've talked about some great ideas, let's get practical — and put what you're learning into action. The Daniel Plan centers around five essential areas of health. In this study you're exploring Fitness, so you can begin by identifying one or two steps you can take to incorporate more movement into your life. Then check out the Food Tip of the Week and the Fitness Move of the Week for some fresh ideas to enrich your journey toward health in those areas. There are also many tips and tools on the danielplan.com website so you can keep growing in all of the Essentials while doing this study. Use or adapt whatever is helpful to you!

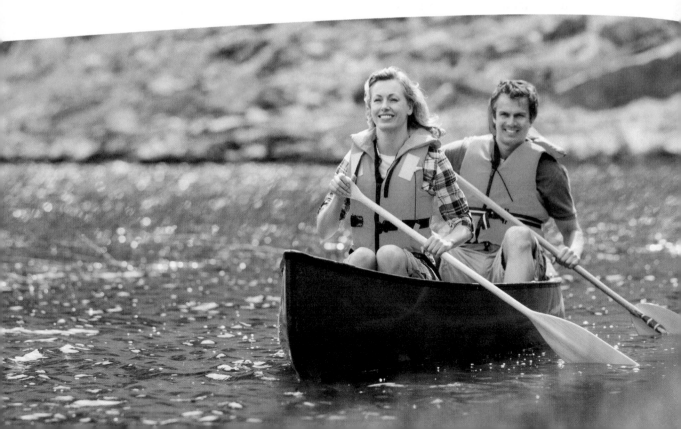

FITNESS
Next Steps

Here are a few suggested activities to help you move forward in becoming Daniel Strong. Check one or two boxes next to the options you'd like to try this week—choose what works for you.

☐ If you didn't identify and write down your big dream during the group meeting, take time this week to do that. Close your eyes and let yourself dream of what you would do to honor God if you were as fit as you could be. Picture yourself fit and doing that. Write your dream on a card or piece of paper.

☐ Post your big dream somewhere you will see it every day. Reread it and let it motivate you. What is the first small step you need to take to head toward that dream?

☐ Find a buddy who will go for walks or to the gym with you. Schedule time to work out together at least once a week for the next few weeks. If you don't have an exercise buddy but want one, what is one small step you can take to find one?

☐ Start a quest for physical activities you enjoy. Page 172 of *The Daniel Plan* book has a list of ideas. Don't hesitate to go after activities you enjoyed as a child. Get a hula hoop, a jump rope, a mini trampoline, or a pair of roller blades or skates. Or play worship music and dance up a storm!

☐ Visit a gym and ask an employee to explain their classes to you. For example, what is Zumba? What level of class are you looking for— something for a beginner or something more advanced? Listen for class ideas that sound like fun to you. Even better: visit a gym where a friend of yours belongs and see if you would enjoy doing a class together.

☐ Try one of The Daniel Plan DVD fitness resources. *The Daniel Plan in Action* DVD contains four 35-minute workouts. *The Daniel Plan in Action: Accelerated* DVD contains six 35-minute and two 45-minute workouts. They are faith-infused and come with a complementary nutrition guide. You can do the workouts on your own or in a group. Ask your church to host a group! For details, see http://store.danielplan.com/fitness-program/.

☐ Sit down with your calendar and find time in your schedule for exercise. Can you schedule ten minutes of brisk walking each day? Can you schedule fifteen minutes twice a day? Be creative, and put exercise into your calendar as an appointment.

☐ Do the Fitness Move of the Week at least three times this week.

☐ Memorize one verse related to Fitness. See the memory verses in the Appendix. You can even recite or meditate on your memory verse while doing the Fitness Move of the Week!

Food Tip
of the Week

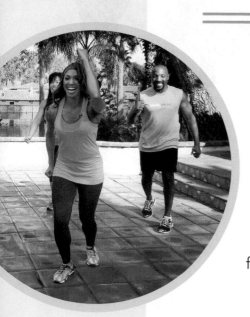

You may have heard the term *superfoods* — nutrient-dense foods that pack extra nutritional punch into every package. Superfoods can be found in fruits and vegetables, seafood like salmon, nuts, seeds, even green tea and dark chocolate. Including superfoods in your diet supports healthy eating and gives you the strength to follow the Fitness Essential principles. This week's food tip shows you how to make a delicious parfait that's full of superfoods. Just click the Food Tip of the Week on your video screen (3 minutes), scan the QR code, or go to daniel plan.com/foodtip.

Fitness Move
of the Week

This week's move is great for burning calories: cross-country skiing with no snow! Just click the Fitness Move of the Week on your video screen (1 minute), use the QR code, or go to danielplan.com/fitnessmove.

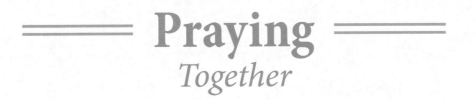

Praying
Together

Because everything we do in our journey toward health depends on God's power, we end each meeting with prayer and encourage group members to pray for each other during the week.

"If you sinful people know how to give good gifts to your children, how much more will your heavenly Father give the Holy Spirit to those who ask him."

Luke 11:13 (NLT)

This week, ask God for power from the Holy Spirit to take a step forward on your journey toward fitness. Each person can offer a one- or two-sentence prayer completing this sentence: "Father, please fill me with your Holy Spirit so that I can _____."

Have someone close with this prayer:

Thank you, Lord, that you give your Holy Spirit for guidance and strength to those who ask. Please fill us with your Spirit so that we can identify movement we enjoy and practice it regularly throughout the week. Please help us overcome our habits of not moving. Please show us what we would be like if we were fit and healthy, and what we could do to honor God if we were like that. Please open our eyes to your big dream for each of us. Please strengthen us with courage and perseverance. Thank you that you are always with us. I pray this in Jesus' name. Amen.

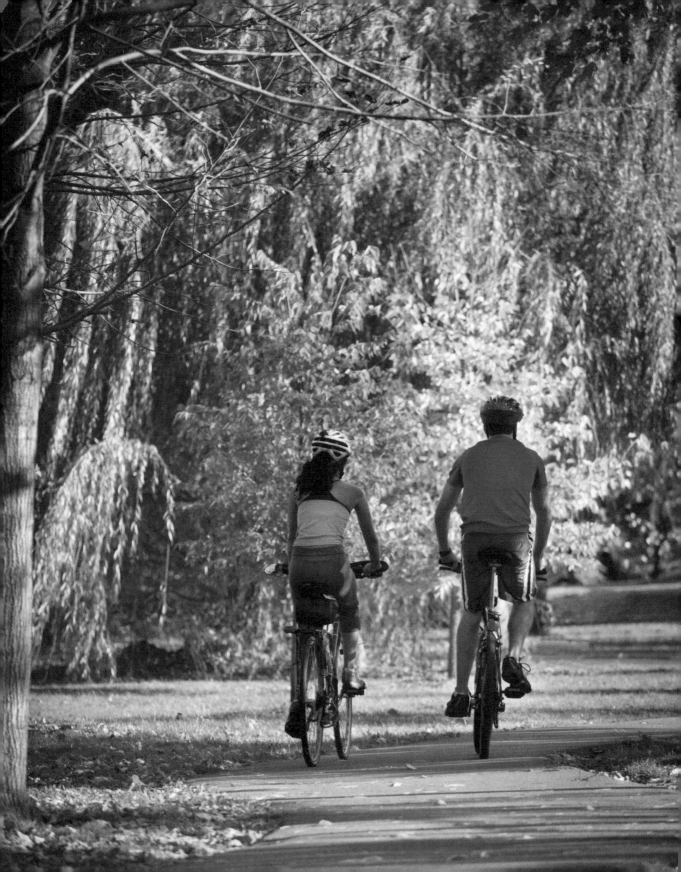

Discover Movement You Enjoy

> "You made my body, Lord; now
> give me sense to heed your laws."
> Psalm 119:73 (TLB)

Sitting has become an actual disease. A whopping 70 percent of Americans are not moving enough to maintain their present health. We each need a plan to incorporate more movement into our days—not just in one workout, but throughout the day. This session will get you started toward just such a plan, moving a couple of minutes here and a couple of minutes there so that you still get your important tasks done but aren't sitting for hours without a break.

COMING
TOGETHER

The other members of your group can be a huge source of support in sustaining healthy changes in your life. Before watching the video, check in with each other about your experiences since the last session. For example:

» Briefly share what Next Steps from Session 1 you completed or tried to complete. Were they helpful? If so, how?

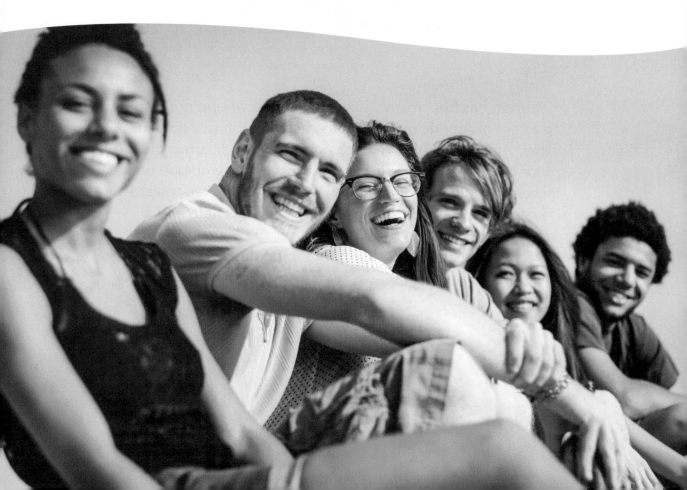

» How did Session 1 affect your relationship with God? With your body?

» Have you been practicing The Daniel Plan in other areas, such as Food? If so, what have you done? What is working well for you? What questions do you have? What encouragement do you need?

LEARNING
TOGETHER

Play the video segment for Session 2. As you watch, use the outline provided to follow along or to take additional notes on anything that stands out to you.

» Seventy percent of Americans are not moving enough just to maintain their present health.

» If you sit for longer than three hours at a time, you shut off an enzyme that is responsible for burning fat. So your body is actually learning to store more fat just because you are seated.

» In the morning while making breakfast, throw in just five minutes of squats, jumping jacks, and marching.

» At work, invite someone for a walking meeting instead of a seated meeting.

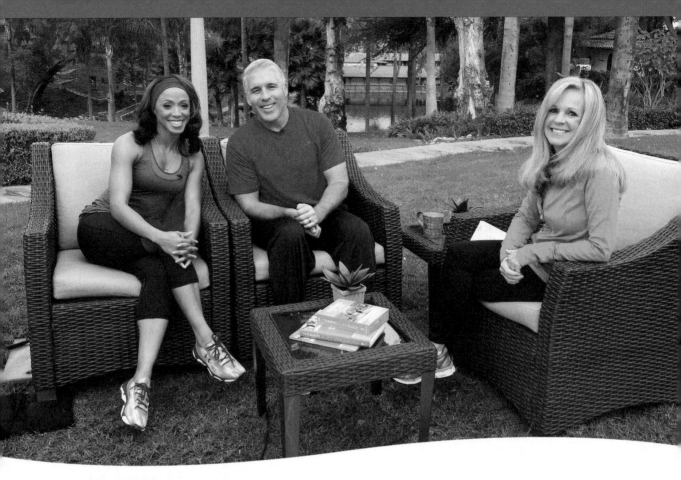

» Park farther from your destination and walk. Take the stairs instead of the elevator.

» Don't separate faith from your workout. You have the body that God created. It is his. You're working on it. So, it's okay to call on him in those moments when caring for your body feels difficult. Ask him for the strength and courage to even start.

» Set an alarm to go off every hour. When the alarm goes off, you move for one to two minutes.

- P is for Prayerful Movements. Stand, place all of your weight on your right foot, and bring your left leg up just a little bit. Raise your hands over your head and look up. Hold this position for thirty seconds, and then switch legs. While you hold, breathe in and out and thank God for your body.

- L is for Lengthening, stretching. Stand and raise your hands over your head. Reach as high as you can and look up. Inhale deeply, taking in God's love and meditating on a verse of Scripture. Lower your hands to your thighs and exhale. Hinge at the waist and let your arms hang. Let your back and hamstrings stretch for thirty seconds. Straighten up slowly, using your abdominal muscles to support your back.

- A is for Aerobic Activity or active sports. Do a minute of jumping jacks.

- Y is for Youthful Strength Training. Press down on the arm of your chair and lift your body for an upper arm workout. Hold for a minute, meditating on a passage of Scripture or worshiping the Lord.

» This week, set a goal for your fitness. Write it down. Make it specific, measurable, and something you can do. For example, "walk one block each day."

GROWING
TOGETHER

Discuss what you learned from the video. Don't feel obliged to answer every question. Select those that most resonate with your group.

 How do you respond to the idea of involving your faith in your fitness, such as by praying for strength and meditating on Scripture while you are moving? In what other ways could you involve your faith with your fitness?

Choose either Isaiah 40:31 or 1 Corinthians 6:19–20, printed below, and tell how it motivates you to get moving. Or share another verse that inspires you.

"Those who hope in the LORD will renew their strength. They will soar on wings like eagles; they will run and not grow weary, they will walk and not be faint."
Isaiah 40:31

"Do you not know that your bodies are temples of the Holy Spirit, who is in you, whom you have received from God? You are not your own; you were bought at a price. Therefore honor God with your bodies."
1 Corinthians 6:19–20

 What can you do to incorporate more movement into your day?

What motivates you to move more during the day? What gets in the way?

 How can you address the obstacles you have identified?

 Talk about possible goals you could set for yourself in the areas of:

» Prayerful movement

» Lengthening

» Aerobic activity

» Youthful strength training

Note: See the 40-Day Fitness Challenge Sample in the Appendix for ideas about goals. Consider committing to the first six days of the challenge.

How can this group support you as you seek to improve your fitness?

What I Want
to Remember

Complete this activity on your own.

» Briefly review the video outline and any notes you took. Review also any notes from the discussion.

» In the space below, write down the most significant thing you gained from this session—from the video or the discussion. You can share it with the group if you wish.

BETTER
TOGETHER

Now that you've talked about some great ideas, let's get practical — and put what you're learning into action. Begin by identifying one or two steps you can take to build your fitness. Then check out the Food Tip of the Week and the Fitness Move of the Week for some fresh ideas to enrich your journey toward health in those areas. Use or adapt whatever is helpful to you!

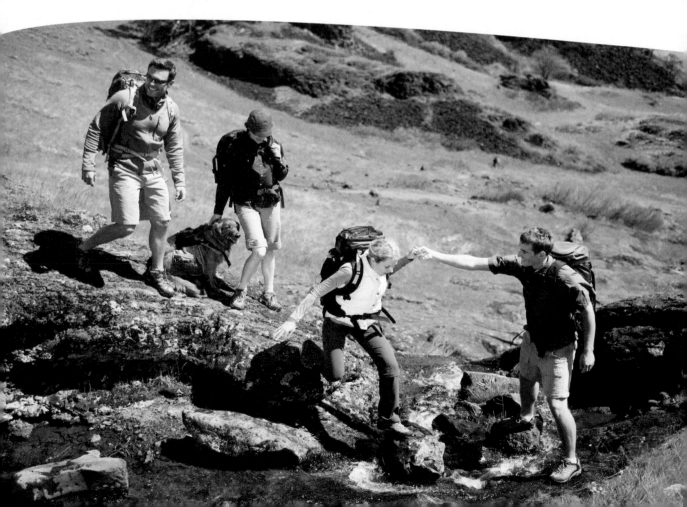

FITNESS
Next Steps

Here are a few suggested activities to help you move forward in becoming Daniel Strong. Check one or two boxes next to the options you'd like to try this week—choose what works for you.

☐ Do the 40-Day Fitness Challenge Sample in the Appendix of this study guide. Will you be at level 1, level 2, or level 3? Better still: team up with a buddy to do the fitness challenge together or to encourage each other as you do the exercises on your own. What encouragement would be most helpful to you?

☐ Get *The Daniel Plan* book to see the rest of the 40-Day Fitness Challenge.

☐ Go for a 20-minute brisk walk three days this week. Better still: get a buddy to go with you.

☐ Get *The Daniel Plan in Action* DVD or *The Daniel Plan in Action: Accelerated* DVD. See http://store.danielplan.com/fitness-program/.

☐ Do the Fitness Move of the Week three days this week, with a day of rest in between.

☐ Set an alarm on your phone to go off every hour. Do two minutes of movement each hour—either prayerful movement, lengthening, aerobic activity, or youthful strength training.

☐ Set your own goal for movement this week. If you've been inactive for more than a few months, start slowly and allow a day of rest between days of exercise (except walking, which can be done every day). Listen to your body so that muscle soreness doesn't become excessive and so that you don't injure yourself.

☐ Memorize the Fitness verse for Session 2. See the memory verses in the Appendix. Post your verse someplace where you will see it often.

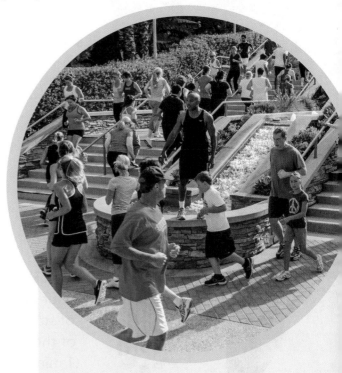

Food Tip
of the Week

Good clean water is essential to our bodies' functioning, yet we often don't get enough. Proper hydration will improve your health. If you find drinking enough water difficult, learn to make flavored waters that taste great and get the job done. Just click the Food Tip of the Week on your video screen (3 minutes), scan the QR code, or go to danielplan.com/foodtip.

Fitness Move
of theWeek

Check out these three moves you can do for your heart and your inner thighs using just a set of stairs. Just click the Fitness Move of the Week on your video screen (1 minute), use the QR code, or go to danielplan.com/fitnessmove.

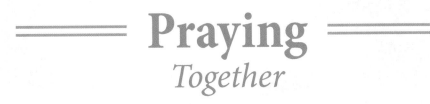

Praying
Together

Because everything we do in our journey toward health depends on God's power, we end each meeting with prayer and encourage group members to pray for each other during the week.

> *"I can do everything through Christ,*
> *who gives me strength."*
> Philippians 4:13 (NLT)

Get into smaller groups of two or three people. Share with your partner(s) the number one thing you need prayer for regarding your fitness. Then pray for your partner(s). Even a sentence is fine. After you've prayed in smaller groups, have someone close with this prayer:

Father, we want to honor you with our bodies. We want to overcome sitting disease by incorporating more movement into our days. You have promised that if we hope in you, you will renew our strength. We want to hope in you this week. We want to rely completely on you for the strength and courage to set and complete our fitness goals. Please fill us with your Spirit to do what we can't do in our own strength. Empower us to walk, run, even soar like eagles. I pray this in Jesus' name. Amen.

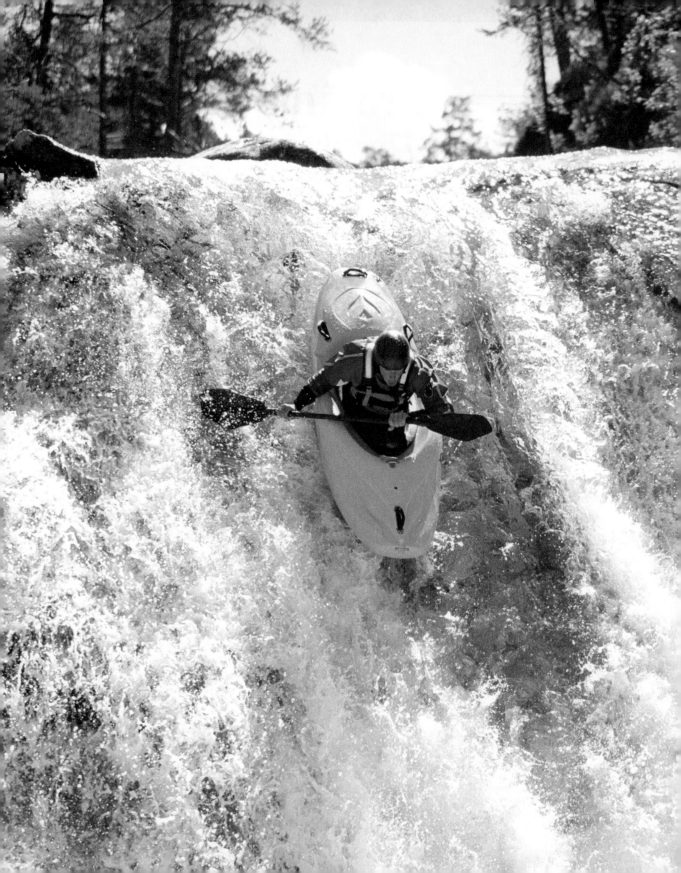

Get a Metabolic Makeover

> "No one hates his own body but feeds and cares for it, just as Christ cares for the church."
> Ephesians 5:29 (NLT)

Your *metabolism* is how your body processes energy. A faster metabolism burns fat while maintaining the body's muscle mass and fluids. The slower your metabolism, the less food you need and the harder it is to lose fat without losing muscle.

If your metabolism is slow, are you stuck with it? The good news is that there are simple things you can do to speed up your metabolism and burn more fat over the course of the day. In this session, you'll learn how to get a metabolic makeover.

COMING
TOGETHER

Before watching the video, check in with each other about your experiences since the last session. For example:

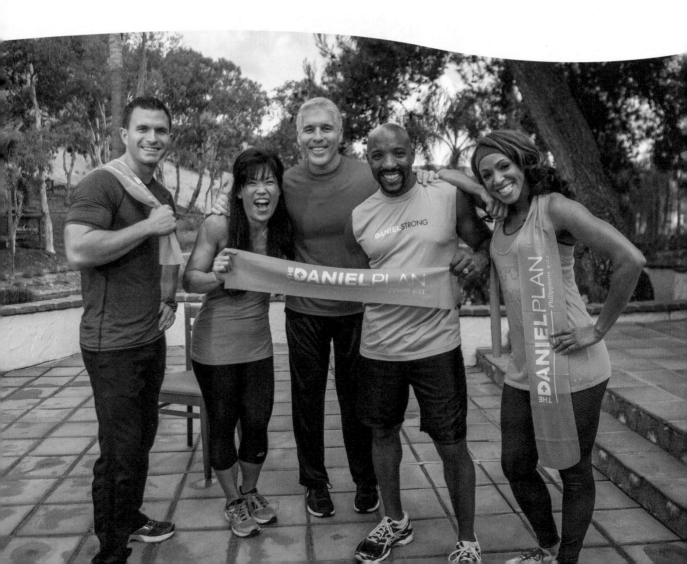

» Briefly share what Next Steps from Session 2 you completed or tried to complete. Were they helpful? If so, how?

» How did Session 2 affect your movement throughout your days this week? How did it affect your ability to connect your faith with your fitness? If you're doing the 40-day challenge, how is it going?

» Have you been practicing The Daniel Plan in other areas, such as Food? If so, what have you done? What is working well for you? What questions do you have? What encouragement do you need?

LEARNING
TOGETHER

AN INTERVIEW WITH Sean Foy

Play the video segment for Session 3. As you watch, use the outline provided to follow along or to take additional notes on anything that stands out to you.

» Your *metabolism* is all the chemical reactions that are occurring in your body. It is how your body processes energy.

» Your *metabolic rate* is the rate at which your body burns or uses energy.

» Many Americans consume the majority of their calories between 6:00 and 10:00 p.m. But our metabolic rate is actually 25 percent slower in the evening.

» In the fat cells of a person who has been on a diet that deprives him or her of nutrients, the lypogenic (fat-storing) enzymes increase by 50 percent, and the lypolytic (fat-burning) enzymes decrease by almost 50 percent. So the person on a diet is telling his or her body to store fat.

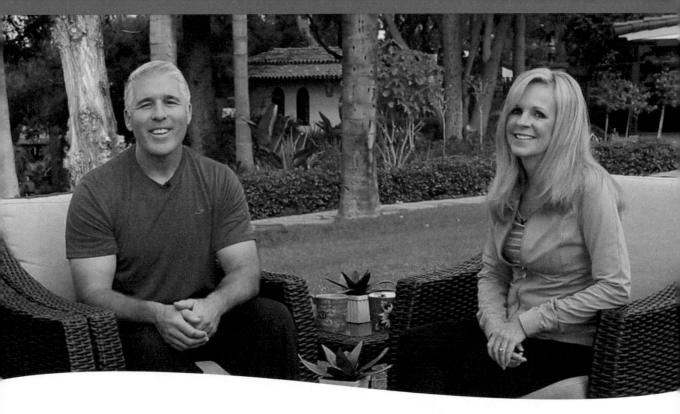

» Four factors influence your metabolism:
  • Basal metabolic rate—the rate at which you burn energy while at rest
  • Lifestyle
  • Exercise
  • Specific dynamic effect—the amount of food you consume

» When you eat, your metabolism increases. Certain foods, such as red pepper and green tea, increase it more. Eating small, frequent meals throughout the day also increases it more than does eating a couple of large meals.

» Our metabolism decreases from 2 to 5 percent every ten years past the age of twenty-five.

» Aerobic exercise is the number one way to increase fat-burning enzymes. Your metabolism is higher after aerobic activity.

» Interval training is moving your body quickly, then slowly, then quickly, then slowly. If you move your body for thirty seconds quickly, then thirty seconds slowly, back and forth, you can burn nine times more body fat than if you move it slowly the whole time.

» Any aerobic activity can be turned into interval training by adding short bursts in which you move as fast as you can for fifteen, thirty, or sixty seconds.

» Even one minute of interval training every hour of your day can significantly increase your metabolism and your health.

» Resistance training builds muscle. The greater your muscle mass, the higher your metabolism, because muscle burns energy.

Note: The 40-Day Fitness Challenge has ideas for starting to build your muscles. See also the workouts in *The Daniel Plan in Action* DVD.

GROWING
TOGETHER

Discuss what you learned from the video. Don't feel obliged to answer every question. Select those that most resonate with your group.

 1   What can we do to boost our metabolic rate?

> *"The LORD gives his people strength.*
> *The LORD blesses them with peace."*
>
> Psalm 29:11 (NLT)

 2   How does diet affect fat-burning enzymes? How does exercise affect them?

"Don't you realize that in a race everyone runs, but only one person gets the prize? So run to win! All athletes are disciplined in their training. They do it to win a prize that will fade away, but we do it for an eternal prize. So I run with purpose in every step. I am not just shadowboxing. I discipline my body like an athlete, training it to do what it should. Otherwise, I fear that after preaching to others I myself might be disqualified."

1 Corinthians 9:24–27 (NLT)

3 In what ways is the information about metabolism and enzymes helpful to you?

4 How does interval training work? Give an example of interval training.

Can you imagine yourself doing interval training? Why or why not?

 Can you imagine yourself doing resistance training two or three times a week? Why or why not?

 What would help you address any barriers you feel toward interval or resistance training?

"The LORD is my strength and shield.
I trust him with all my heart. He helps me,
and my heart is filled with joy."

Psalm 28:7 (NLT)

What I Want
to Remember

Complete this activity on your own.

» Briefly review the video outline and any notes you took. Review also any notes from the discussion.

» In the space below, write down the most significant thing you gained from this session—from the video or the discussion. You can share it with the group if you wish.

BETTER
TOGETHER

Now that you've talked about some great ideas, let's get practical — and put what you're learning into action. Begin by identifying one or two steps you can take to build your fitness. Then check out the Food Tip of the Week and the Fitness Move of the Week for some fresh ideas to enrich your journey toward health in those areas. Use or adapt whatever is helpful to you!

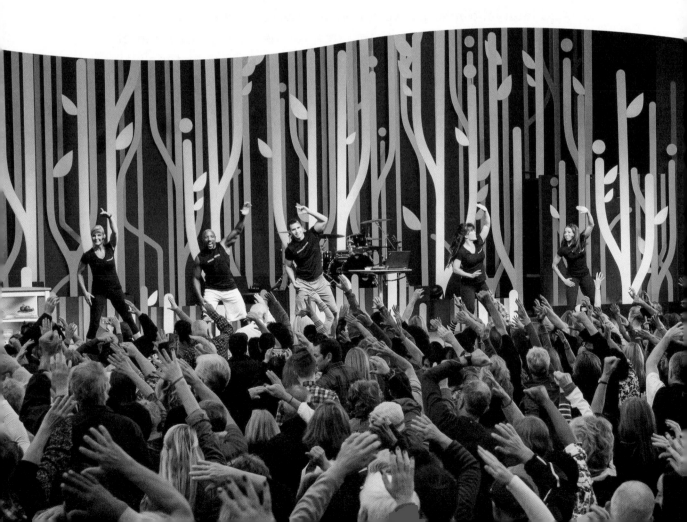

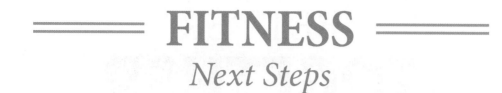

FITNESS
Next Steps

Here are a few suggested activities to help you experiment with interval and resistance training. Check one or two boxes next to the options you'd like to try this week—choose what works for you.

- ☐ Do interval training for one to two minutes every hour throughout your day. Set an alarm to remind you.

- ☐ Add interval training to your aerobic workouts three days a week. If you're walking for twenty minutes, for instance, put a burst of energy into walking as fast as you can for one minute, then walk four minutes at your regular brisk pace. Do that four times in twenty minutes. If you're walking with a buddy, make those bursts of faster walking a friendly competition to spur each other on.

- ☐ Do at least ten minutes (or twenty if you're ready for it) of resistance training at least twice during the week. See the 40-Day Fitness Challenge or danielplan.com for ideas.

- ☐ Sign up with a personal trainer or get a friend who can guide you in resistance training that is appropriate for you. Be sure to choose a trainer who knows how to work with people of your age and fitness level.

☐ Try a class at the gym that mixes resistance training with aerobic activity. Ask one of the staff to tell you which classes do that. Choose a class that is right for your fitness level.

☐ Memorize a verse for this week, and then meditate on it while you do the Fitness Move of the Week. See the memory verses in the Appendix.

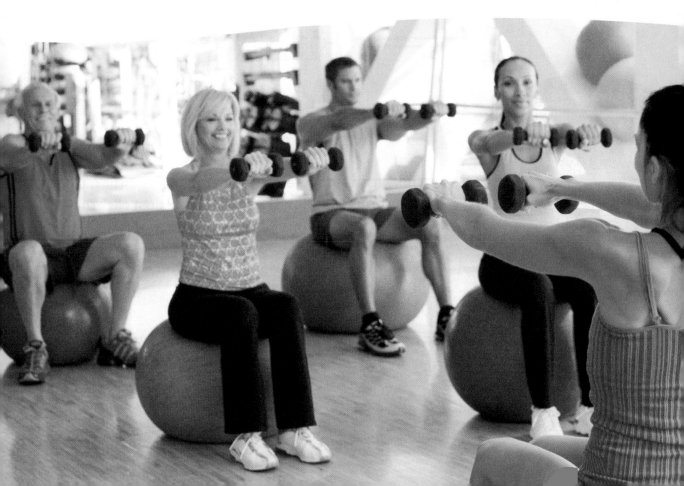

Food Tip
of the Week

Want to learn how to rehydrate and refuel after you work out? Learn a great smoothie recipe. Just click the Food Tip of the Week on your video screen (3 minutes), scan the QR code, or go to danielplan.com/foodtip.

Fitness Move
of the Week

Take a one-minute break in your day of sitting to do something fun: shadow boxing! Just click the Fitness Move of the Week on your video screen (1 minute), use the QR code, or go to danielplan.com/fitnessmove.

Praying
Together

Because everything we do in our journey toward health depends on God's power, we end each meeting with prayer and encourage group members to pray for each other during the week.

"Therefore, I urge you, brothers and sisters, in view of God's mercy, to offer your bodies as a living sacrifice, holy and pleasing to God— this is your true and proper worship."

Romans 12:1

Get into smaller groups of two or three people. Share with your partner(s) the number one thing you need prayer for regarding your fitness. Then pray for your partner(s). Have someone close with this prayer:

Lord, our bodies truly are fearfully and wonderfully made. We are in awe of the way you have designed our bodies to follow laws that you have built into them. Please help us understand those laws and so to live wisely, in ways that make our bodies flourish. Please help us understand how metabolism works so that we can increase our metabolic rate and burn the fuel we consume. Give us the courage to try something new and the perseverance to keep on with our fitness goals. Help us recover our childhood sense of play. Remind us of our big dreams so that they motivate us. You are our strength every day, and we want to rely utterly on you. I pray this in Jesus' name. Amen.

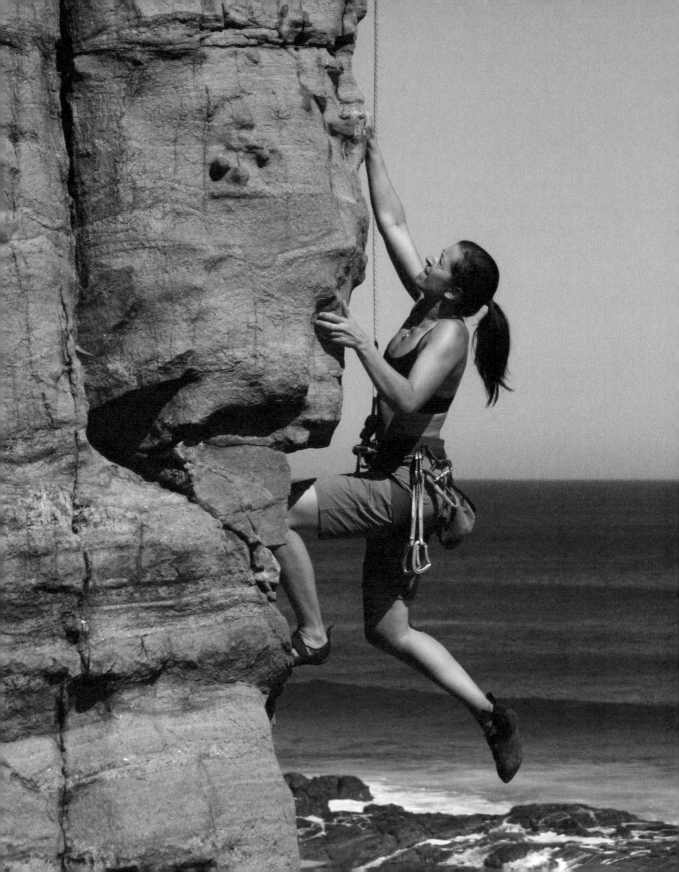

Breaking through the Wall

> "Be patient, then, brothers and sisters, until the Lord's coming. See how the farmer waits for the land to yield its valuable crop, patiently waiting for the autumn and spring rains."
> James 5:7

In a culture of quick texts, overnight shipping, and microwave ovens, we are used to expecting fast results. But with fitness, results take time. Building muscles takes time. In fact, changing habits takes time. Maybe you are all in with the 40-Day Fitness Challenge, or maybe you're still deciding what you think about what you've learned about fitness. Maybe you started off toward your fitness goals with great intentions, but the realities of the rest of your life are pressing in on you. That's normal. Sooner or later in the process of change, we all hit walls that seem to have no way around them and no way through. In this final session we'll address four common walls people hit when they try to build their fitness, and we'll look at how the change process really works.

COMING
TOGETHER

Before watching the video, check in with each other about your experiences since the last session. For example:

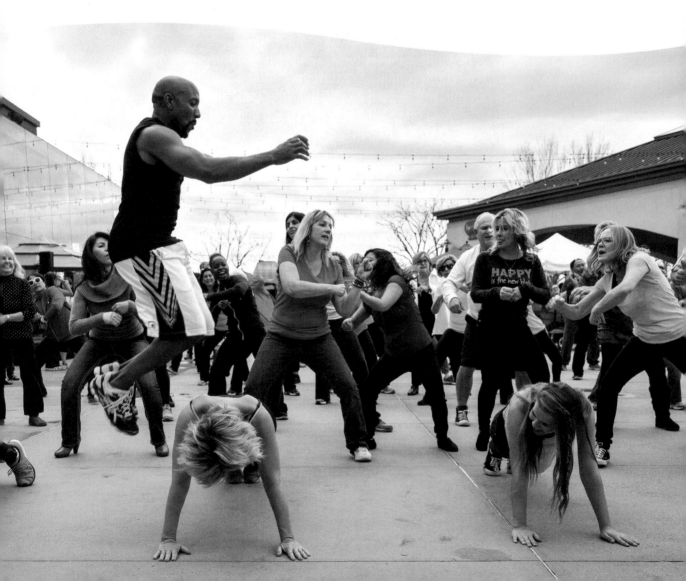

» Briefly share what Next Steps from Session 3 you completed or tried to complete. Were they helpful? If so, how?

» How did Session 3 affect your movement throughout the day during this past week? If you're doing the 40-day challenge, how is it going?

» How have you been relying on God to reach your fitness goals? What have you been saying to God?

» Have you been practicing The Daniel Plan in other areas, such as Food? If so, what have you done? What is working well for you? What questions do you have? What encouragement do you need?

LEARNING
TOGETHER

AN INTERVIEW WITH Sean Foy AND Basheerah Ahmad

Play the video segment for Session 4. As you watch, use the outline provided to follow along or to take additional notes on anything that stands out to you.

» The top barriers people face in pursuing a healthy, active lifestyle are:

  * Time

  * Motivation—what can motivate us to maintain our healthy, active lifestyle over the long run, especially when our weight hits a plateau?

  * Boredom—we get tired of doing the same thing over and over

  * Discomfort with making our health a priority

» It's crucial to set a goal that is stronger and longer-term than the desire to fit into a particular dress or pair of pants. We need a big dream like the one we discussed in Session 1.

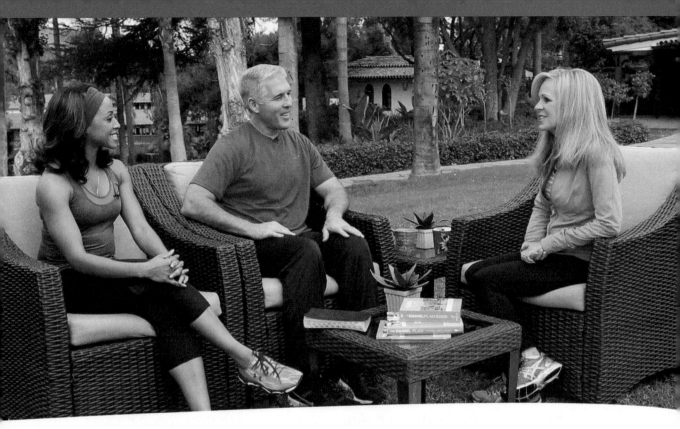

» We need to have some level of faith in our ability to achieve our goal. It can't be so unrealistic that we lose hope of attaining it.

» We need to see the value of taking care of our bodies so that we are able to care for others. We need to not feel guilty about the time it takes to care for ourselves.

» We need to be content with where we are on the journey toward fitness. We need to avoid comparing ourselves with others.

» If we nurture our inner lives through things like prayer and journaling, we will be drawn to nurture our bodies through healthy eating and exercise.

» There are five stages that we all go through when we change:

- Stage one is *not thinking about changing*. We are locked into denial, rationalizing our behavior because we want to stay there.

- Stage two is *thinking about changing*. We read a book; we gather information. This is important to the change process. However, we can get stuck there, chronically thinking about changing tomorrow but never actually doing it. Alternatively, we can take specific steps to move to the next stage.

- Stage three is *planning*. It is sitting down and writing out our goals, and creating an action step that is specific and measurable. We write down our big dream, and we set the date for our first walk.

- Stage four is *action*. We jump in and start exercising. We get our shoes on and start to walk, or we go for a session with a personal trainer.

- Stage five is *maintenance*. This is actually staying with the new behavior for at least six months. Support is crucial to stage five. We need buddies to support us.

» Throw away your scale if weighing yourself is demotivating. If you are eating right and exercising, then the scale is not giving you helpful information.

» Two good long-term motivations for exercising are physical and emotional health. Not only does exercise address heart and blood sugar problems, but it also lifts mood and overcomes anxiety, depression, and stress.

» In those moments when we feel we can't go any further, turning to God's grace and throwing our reliance wholly on him is crucial.

GROWING
TOGETHER

Discuss what you learned from the video. Don't feel obliged to answer every question. Select those that most resonate with your group.

 What did you hear in the video that had the most impact on you?

 Recall the five stages of change. At which stage are you in the process of changing to a healthy fitness lifestyle?

 What would help you move to the next stage of change?

"We also pray that you will be strengthened with all his glorious power so you will have all the endurance and patience you need. May you be filled with joy, always thanking the Father."
Colossians 1:11–12 (NLT)

What benefits would there be for you, your family, and your friends if you were to move more on a regular basis? Start with personal benefits, but also think about how others in your life would benefit. Have someone in the group volunteer to write down all of the ideas the group can generate and then email the list to the group.

 What barriers will you need to contend with in order to exercise regularly and incorporate movement throughout your day?

 What are some potential solutions to those barriers? Have someone in the group write down the solutions you come up with and later email them to the group. Try to address at least two of the following barriers (or other barriers) for each person in the group:

» Time

» Motivation

» Boredom

» Prioritizing health

"As you know, we count as blessed those who have persevered. You have heard of Job's perseverance and have seen what the Lord finally brought about. The Lord is full of compassion and mercy."

James 5:11

 What are the most valuable things you have gotten out of this Fitness study? What will you take with you? What goal do you have to continue moving forward? How can the group help?

What I Want
to Remember

Complete this activity on your own.

» Briefly review the video outline and any notes you took. Review also any notes from the discussion.

» In the space below, write down the most significant thing you gained from this session — from the video or the discussion. You can share it with the group if you wish.

BETTER
TOGETHER

Now that you've talked about some great ideas, let's get practical—and put what you're learning into action. Begin by identifying one or two steps you can take to build your fitness. Then check out the Food Tip of the Week and the Fitness Move of the Week for some fresh ideas to enrich your journey toward health in those areas. Use or adapt whatever is helpful to you!

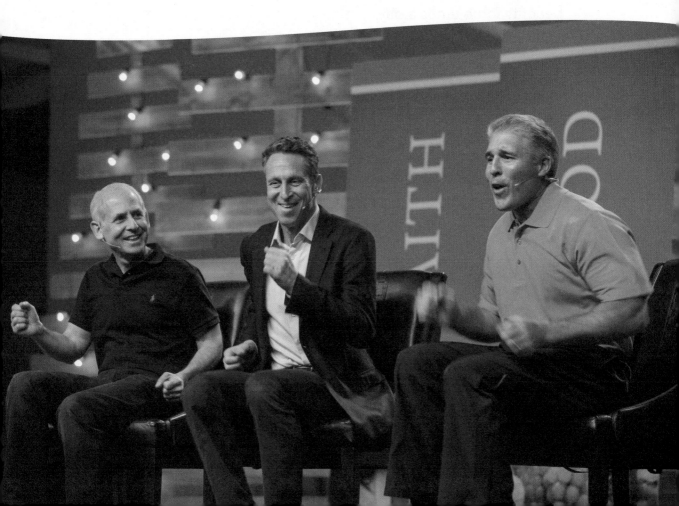

FITNESS
Next Steps

Here are a few suggested activities to help you move forward in maintaining a lifestyle of fitness over the long haul. Check one or two boxes next to the options you'd like to try this week — choose what works for you.

☐ Write on one side of a 3 x 5 card all of the benefits to you, your family, and your friends if you were to move and exercise regularly. Write on the other side of the card the barriers you would need to contend with in order to move and exercise regularly. Write as much as you can on the solutions to those barriers. Commit to reading the benefits three times a day.

☐ Drill down on the solutions to your barriers. Write down ideas as they occur to you. For instance, what are some creative solutions to the barrier of time? If you go all out with movement for 2 minutes an hour, in a 14-hour day you will have moved for 28 minutes. Can you add in a 10-minute walk? Another way to approach the time problem is to build movement into your current activities by having walking meetings or marching while you're on the phone. If there's time in your day when you're watching TV or amusing yourself on the Internet, can you shift that to time spent moving?

☐ Maybe your main barrier is boredom. If so, what can you do to build variety into your movement life? How can you identify movement you enjoy? What is one step you can take toward doing that? Or what is one step you can take toward finding a buddy to exercise with? Get *The Daniel Plan* book and see how many ideas for movement there are. Get all five of the video study guides in this series, view all of the Fitness Moves of the Week, and identify five moves that look fun enough to do regularly throughout your week. Or branch out to a type of class at the gym you haven't tried before.

☐ If motivation is a barrier for you, revisit your big dream. Would it help you to read your dream every day? If your dream isn't motivating you to move enough, spend some time in prayer, asking God to show you who you could be if your body were fit, and what you could do to honor him with a fit body. Keep persistently praying about this until God shows you something that will motivate you. Open your eyes and ears throughout the day to possible answers to that prayer. What can't you do now that you could do with a fit body? What are you too tired for, or too much in pain for, or too out of shape for?

☐ Maybe you weren't ready to start the 40-Day Fitness Challenge a couple of weeks ago, but now you are. Go for it! Ask someone in your group to cheer you on for the next forty days.

☐ Memorize a verse this week to stay encouraged. See the memory verses in the Appendix.

Food Tip
of the Week

Smart snacking keeps your blood sugar stable with nutritious choices while keeping your energy up. This week's food tip shows you how to make something easy that tastes fantastic: no-bake power bites. Just click the Food Tip of the Week on your video screen (3 minutes), scan the QR code, or go to danielplan.com/foodtip.

Fitness Move
of the Week

Anytime, anywhere, you can do some interval training by speed skating without skates. To learn how, just click the Fitness Move of the Week on your video screen (1 minute), use the QR code, or go to danielplan.com/fitnessmove.

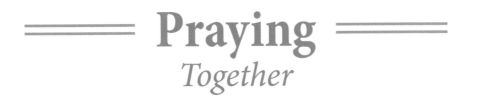

Praying
Together

Because everything we do in our journey toward health depends on God's power, we end each meeting with prayer and encourage group members to pray for each other during the week.

"Rejoice always, pray continually, give thanks in all circumstances; for this is God's will for you in Christ Jesus."
1 Thessalonians 5:16 – 18

This week, focus on gratitude. Offer God one- and two-sentence prayers of thanksgiving for what he is doing in your lives. Thank him for what you have learned about fitness and for giving you the strength to take the steps you've taken. Thank him for what this group has meant to you.
Have someone close with this prayer:

Father, thank you for making us with bodies. Thank you for these specific bodies that we have. No matter how old they are, and even if they have permanent limitations, we know they are your precious gift to us, and the way they work is marvelous. Thank you for everything you've taught us about how to take care of these bodies that you have entrusted to us. Thank you for what we've learned about what motivates us, for the big dreams you have given each of us—the things we could do with fit bodies to honor you. Thank you for teaching us about aerobic activity and stretching and strength training and interval training. Thank you that even small steps like two-minute bursts of activity are significant to you. Thank you for the encouragement we've gotten from others in this group. Please show us what Next Steps you have for each of us in the area of fitness. Please empower us through your Holy Spirit to overcome the barriers of time, motivation, boredom, lack of value, and any other barrier that stands in the way of our living the way you are calling us to live. Please give us perseverance, endurance, and patience. I pray this in Jesus' name. Amen.

Appendix

40-Day Fitness Challenge Sample

To help you begin your fitness journey, chapter 9 of *The Daniel Plan* book offers the 40-Day Fitness Challenge. It contains suggested daily exercises — what we like to call the "play of the day" — to help you reach your fitness goals. The intent is for you to become Daniel Strong by exercising six days of the week for 40 days.

The first week of the fitness challenge (six days, because the seventh is a day for rest) is given here as a sample. We encourage you to get the book and complete the remainder of the 40 days. You will see how easy it can be to move your body with an easy-to-follow plan. The 40-day challenge gives you a template that allows you to exchange exercises you prefer in place of those that are suggested.

DANIEL STRONG LEVELS

You can select from three levels of exercise, depending on where you are at with fitness right now.

» **Daniel Strong 1** is recommended for individuals who are beginning, are restarting, or have time constraints. Recommended movements in this level are designed to help you slowly and safely incorporate exercise into a busy life.

» **Daniel Strong 2** is recommended for individuals who have been exercising occasionally or have the ability and desire to spend a little more time exercising. Exercises at this level are designed to help you step it up a bit, progressively challenging you to become Daniel Strong.

» **Daniel Strong 3** is designed for individuals who are already active and ready for an advanced challenge. The routines found here will take your fitness to another level. Level 3 exercises are online; go to danielplan.com for more information.

SUBSTITUTIONS

In place of any of the exercises listed in the sample plan below, you can substitute others from *The Daniel Plan* book, from danielplan.com, or your favorite activities. Page numbers for substitute exercises in the book are given below.

DAY 1 ·

Perform the following activities (or exchange with other aerobic activities found on page 172 or on danielplan.com).

LEVEL 1

Aerobic: Go for a 10-to-20-minute brisk walk.

Stretch: Standing neck stretches; pray or meditate while doing these. Perform this stretch for 10 to 15 seconds to each side at your desk or when at home throughout your day. (See illustration on page 280.)

LEVEL 2

Aerobic: Go for a 20-to-30-minute power walk, walk/jog, interval training, or jog.

Stretch: Complete

- ☐ Standing forward shoulder reach
- ☐ Lunge and bend
- ☐ Walking high kicks

Perform each stretch or movement (see illustrations on pages 280–81) for 10 to 15 seconds each side (or 5 times for each side of your body) before and/or after your aerobic exercise or throughout your day at work or home. Thank God for the blessing of a body that moves.

DAY 2 ·

Perform the following activities (or exchange with other strength activities found on pages 174–75 or at danielplan.com).

LEVEL 1

Strength: Perform one set of 8 to 10 repetitions (or as many as you can do):

☐ Squats
☐ Desk or modified push-ups

(See illustrations on page 282.)

LEVEL 2

Strength: Perform as many repetitions as you can of each exercise below in 20 seconds. Then rest 10 seconds in between each exercise. Once you have completed all exercises, rest for a full 2 minutes. Complete an additional set for a total of two sets:

☐ Overhead squats: 20 seconds/10 seconds rest
☐ Run in place: 20 seconds/10 seconds rest
☐ Military push-ups: 20 seconds/10 seconds rest
☐ Run in place: 20 seconds/10 seconds rest
☐ Front lunges (alternating sides): 20 seconds/10 seconds rest
☐ Elbow plank: 20 seconds/10 seconds rest
☐ Run in place: 20 seconds/rest

(See illustrations on pages 282–83.)

DAY 3 ···

Perform the following activities (or exchange with other activities found on page 172 or on danielplan.com).

LEVEL 1

Aerobic: Go for a 10-to-20-minute bike ride or walk.

Stretch:

☐ Standing neck stretches

☐ Standing shoulder rolls

Complete each movement for 10 seconds to each side (or 5 to 10 times for each shoulder) at your desk or when at home throughout your day. (See illustration on page 280.) Pray or meditate on Scripture during these loosening movements.

LEVEL 2

Aerobic: Go for a 20-to-30-minute power walk, walk/jog, interval training, or jog.

Stretch:

☐ Standing forward shoulder reach

☐ Lunge and bend

☐ Walking high kicks

Perform each stretch or movement for 10 to 15 seconds on each side (or 5 to 10 times each side) before or after your aerobic exercise or throughout your day at work or home. (See illustrations on pages 280–81.) Pray or meditate on Scripture during these loosening movements.

DAY 4 ···

Perform the following activities (or exchange with other activities found on pages 174–75 or on danielplan.com).

LEVEL 1

Strength: Perform one set of 8 to 10 repetitions (or as many as you can do):

☐ Squats

☐ Desk or modified push-ups

☐ Desk or modified planks, hold for 10 seconds

(See illustrations on page 282.)

LEVEL 2

Strength: Perform as many repetitions as you can of each exercise below in 20 seconds. Then rest 10 seconds in between each exercise. Once you have completed all exercises, rest for a full 2 minutes. Complete an additional set for a total of two sets.

☐ Overhead squats: 20 seconds/10 seconds rest

☐ Power skipping: 20 seconds/10 seconds rest

☐ Push-ups: 20 seconds/10 seconds rest

☐ Walking lunges: 20 seconds/10 seconds rest

☐ Power skipping: 20 seconds/10 seconds rest

☐ Elbow plank: 20 seconds/10 seconds rest

☐ Power skipping: 20 seconds/rest

(See illustrations on pages 282–84.)

DAY 5 ··

Perform the following activities (or exchange with other activities found on page 172 or on danielplan.com).

LEVEL 1

Aerobic: Go for a 10-to-20-minute brisk walk.

Stretch:

- ☐ Standing shoulder rolls
- ☐ Standing alternating toe touches

Complete each movement 5 to 10 times (see illustrations on pages 280–81), and thank God for your health as you hold each stretch.

LEVEL 2

Aerobic: Go for a 20-to-30-minute power walk, walk/jog, interval training, or jog.

Stretch:

- ☐ Standing forward shoulder reach
- ☐ Lunge and bend
- ☐ Walking high kicks
- ☐ Elbow to foot lunge

Perform each stretch or movement for 10 to 15 seconds on each side (or 5 to 10 times each side) before or after your aerobic exercise or throughout your day at work or home. (See illustrations on pages 280–81.) Thank God for your health as you hold each stretch.

DAY 6 ···

Perform the following activities (or exchange with other activities found on pages 174–75 or on danielplan.com).

LEVEL 1

Strength: Perform one set of 8 to 10 repetitions (or as many as you can do):

☐ Squats

☐ Desk or modified push-ups

☐ Desk or modified plank, hold for 10 to 15 seconds

(See illustrations on page 282.)

LEVEL 2

Strength: Perform as many repetitions as you can of each exercise below in 15 seconds. Then rest 15 seconds in between each exercise. Once you have completed all exercises, rest for a full 2 minutes. Complete an additional set for a total of two sets:

☐ Overhead squats: 15 seconds/15 seconds rest

☐ Toe touches: 15 seconds/15 seconds rest

☐ Push-ups: 15 seconds/15 seconds rest

☐ Toe touches: 15 seconds/15 seconds rest

☐ Walking lunges: 15 seconds/15 seconds rest

☐ Toe touches: 15 seconds/15 seconds rest

☐ Side plank: 15 seconds/15 seconds rest

☐ Toe touches: 15 seconds/15 seconds rest

(See illustrations on pages 282–83.)

STRETCHING-LOOSENING EXERCISES

Neck stretch chin to chest: Slowly begin to lower your neck down by lowering your chin down to your chest and hold for 10 to 15 seconds.

Neck stretch ear to shoulder: Lower your right ear toward your right shoulder. Hold. Lower your left ear toward your left shoulder. Hold.

Neck rotation: Slowly turn your head to the right. Your chin will be close to your right shoulder. Hold. Slowly turn your head to the left. Your chin will be close to your left shoulder. Hold.

Standing forward shoulder reach: Reach your arms behind your back and interlace your fingers. Lift your shoulders up toward your ears, and lift your hands away from your back. Slowly bend forward at the waist, keeping your back flat, not rounded. Continue bending forward, and lift your hands over your head as far forward as comfortable. At a full stretch, you will feel tension in your hamstrings and in your shoulders.

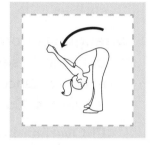

Shoulder rolls: Stand with your arms hanging straight down. Shrug both shoulders forward and up. Roll the shoulders back and down. Make big circles while keeping the head straight.

Alternating toe touches: Stand with your feet spread as far apart as comfortably possible. Then lean forward toward one leg and try to reach your foot or until you feel a comfortable stretch in your lower back and hamstrings. Now try to touch the other foot with the opposite arm.

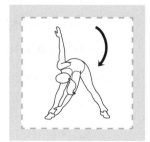

Lunge and bend: Stand tall with your arms hanging at your sides. Step forward with your right leg, and lower your body until your right knee is bent at about 90 degrees. As you lunge, reach over your head with your left arm and bend your torso to your right.

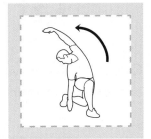

Walking high kick: Stand tall with arms hanging at your sides. Keeping your knee straight, kick your right leg up and reach with your left arm out to meet it as you simultaneously take a step forward. (Imagine that you're a British soldier. As soon as your right foot touches the floor, repeat the movement with your left foot and right arm.)

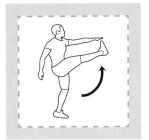

Elbow to foot lunge: Brace your core and lunge forward with your right leg. As you lunge, lean forward at your hips and place your left hand on the floor so it's even with your right foot. Place your right elbow next to the instep of your right foot (or as close as you can), and hold. Next, rotate your torso up and toward the right, reaching as high as you comfortably can with your right hand. Repeat with your left leg and left arm.

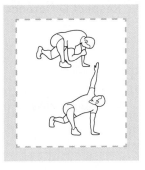

Group Guidelines

Our goal: To provide a safe environment where participants experience authentic community and spiritual growth.

OUR VALUES	
Group Attendance	To give priority to the group meeting. We will call or email if we will be late or absent.
Safe Environment	To help create a safe place where people can be heard and feel loved.
Respect Differences	To be gentle and gracious to people with different spiritual maturity, personal opinions, or personalities. Remember we are all works in progress!
Confidentiality	To keep anything that is shared strictly confidential and within the group, and to avoid sharing information about those outside the group.
Encouragement for Growth	We want to spiritually multiply our life by serving others with our God-given gifts.
Rotating Hosts/Leaders and Homes	To encourage different people to host the group in their homes, and to rotate the responsibility of facilitating each meeting.

We have found that groups thrive when they talk about expectations up front and come into agreement on some of the following details.

Refreshments/mealtimes _____

Child care _____

When we will meet (day of week) _____

Where we will meet (place) _____

We will begin at (time) _____ and end at _____

We will look for a compatible time to attend a worship service together.

Our primary worship service time will be _____

Leadership 101

Congratulations! You have responded to the call to help shepherd Jesus' flock. There are few other tasks in the family of God that surpass the contribution you will be making. As you prepare to lead, whether it is one session or four, here are a few thoughts to keep in mind. We encourage you to read these and review them with each new discussion leader before he or she leads.

1. **Remember that you are not alone.** God knows everything about you, and he knew that you would be asked to lead your group. It is common for leaders to feel that they are not ready to lead. Moses, Solomon, Jeremiah, Timothy—they all were reluctant to lead. God promises, "Never will I leave you; never will I forsake you" (Hebrews 13:5). You will be blessed as you serve.

2. **Don't try to do it alone.** Pray right now for God to help you build a healthy leadership team. If you can enlist a co-leader to help you lead the group, you will find your experience to be much richer. That person might take half the group in a second discussion circle if your group is as large as ten people or more. Your co-leader might lead the prayer time or handle the hosting tasks, welcoming people and getting them refreshments. This is your chance to involve as many people as you can in building a healthy group. All you have to do is call and ask people to help; you'll be surprised at the response.

3. **Just be yourself.** God wants you to use your unique gifts and temperament. Don't try to do things exactly like another leader; do them in a way that fits you! Just admit it when you don't have an answer, and apologize when you make a mistake. Your group will love you for it, and you'll sleep better at night.

4. **Prepare for your meeting ahead of time.** Review the session, view the video, and write down your responses to each question. If paper and pens are needed, such as for gathering group members' names and email addresses (see "Coming Together" in Session 1), be sure you have the necessary supplies. Think about which "Next Steps" you will do.

    If you're leading Session 1, look over the Group Guidelines and be ready to review them with the group. If child care will be an issue for your group, for example, be prepared to talk about options. Some groups have the adults share the cost of a babysitter (or two) to care for children in a different part of the house where the adults are meeting. Other groups use one home for the kids and another for the adults. A third idea is to rotate the responsibility of caring for the children in the same home or one nearby.

5. **Pray for your group members by name.** Before you begin your session, go around the room in your mind and pray for each member. You may want to review the group's prayer list at least once a week. Ask God to use your time together to work in the heart of each person uniquely. Expect God to lead you to whomever he wants you to encourage or challenge in a special way.

6. **When you ask a question, be patient.** Read each question aloud and wait for someone to respond. Sometimes people need a moment or two of silence to think about the question, and if silence doesn't bother you, it won't bother anyone else. After someone responds, affirm the response with a simple "thanks" or "good job." Then ask, "How about somebody else?" or "Would someone who hasn't shared like to add anything?" Be sensitive to new people or reluctant members who aren't ready to participate yet. If you give them a safe setting, they will open up over time. Don't go around the circle and have everyone answer every question. Your goal is a conversation in which the group members talk to each other in a natural way.

7. **Break up into small groups each week or people won't stay.** If your group has more than eight people, we strongly encourage you to have the group gather sometimes in discussion circles of three or four people during the "Growing Together" section of the study. With a greater opportunity to talk in a small circle, people will connect more with the study, apply more quickly what they are learning, and ultimately get more out of it. A small circle also encourages a quiet person to participate and tends to minimize the effect of a more vocal or dominant member. It can also help people feel more loved in your group. When you gather again at the end of the section, you can have one person summarize the highlights from each circle.

   Small circles are also helpful during prayer time. People who are not accustomed to praying aloud will feel more comfortable trying it with just two or three others. Also, prayer requests won't take as much time, so circles will have more time to actually pray. When you gather back with the whole group, you can have one person from each circle briefly update everyone on the prayer requests.

8. **One final challenge for new leaders:** Before your opportunity to lead, look up each of the four passages listed below. Read each one as a devotional exercise to help equip you with a shepherd's heart. If you do this, you will be more than ready for your first meeting.

   Matthew 9:36
   1 Peter 5:2 – 4
   Psalm 23
   Ezekiel 34:11 – 16

   For additional tips and resources, go to danielplan.com/tools.

Memory Verses

SESSION 1

"All glory to God, who is able, through his mighty power at work within us, to accomplish infinitely more than we might ask or think."

Ephesians 3:20 (NLT)

SESSION 2

"Those who hope in the LORD will renew their strength. They will soar on wings like eagles; they will run and not grow weary, they will walk and not be faint."

Isaiah 40:31

SESSION 3

"The LORD is my strength and shield. I trust him with all my heart. He helps me, and my heart is filled with joy."

Psalm 28:7 (NLT)

SESSION 4

"We also pray that you will be strengthened with all his glorious power so you will have all the endurance and patience you need. May you be filled with joy, always thanking the Father."

Colossians 1:11 – 12 (NLT)

About the Contributors

GUEST SPEAKERS

Sean Foy is an internationally renowned authority on fitness, weight management, and healthy living. As an author, exercise physiologist, behavioral coach, and speaker, Sean has earned the reputation as "America's Fast Fitness Expert." With an upbeat and sensible approach to making fitness happen, he's taken the message of "simple moves" fitness all over the world. Sean is the author of *Fitness That Works, Walking 4 Wellness, The Burst Workout,* and a contributing author *The Daniel Plan.* (Sean also served on the Fitness Team for this study.)

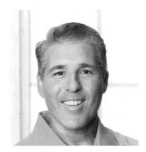

Basheerah Ahmad is a well-known celebrity fitness expert, with a heart for serving God's people. Whether it be through television appearances (*Dr. Phil, The Doctors*), writing fitness and nutrition books, speaking publicly about health, or teaching classes in under-served communities, Basheerah has dedicated her life to improving the health of people everywhere. She has a MS in Exercise Science and numerous certifications in fitness and nutrition. She was a lead fitness instructor for *The Daniel Plan in Action* fitness video series. (Basheerah also served on the Fitness Team for this study.)

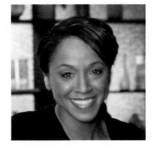

Dee Eastman is the Founding Director of The Daniel Plan that has helped over 15,000 people lose 260,000 pounds in the first year alone. Dee completed her education in Health Science with an emphasis in long-term lifestyle change. Her experience in corporate wellness and ministry has fueled her passion to help people transform their health while drawing closer to God. She coauthored the *Doing Life Together* Bible study series and was a contributing author of *The Daniel Plan.*

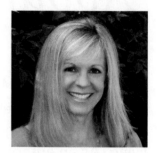

SIGNATURE CHEFS

Sally Cameron is a professional chef, author, recipe developer, educator, certified health coach, and one of the contributors to *The Daniel Plan Cookbook*. Sally's passion is to inspire people to create great-tasting meals at home using healthy ingredients and easy techniques. Sally is the publisher of the popular food blog, *A Food Centric Life*. She holds a culinary degree from The Art Institute and health coaching certification from The Institute for Integrative Nutrition.

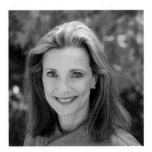

Jenny Ross is the internationally recognized chef, author, educator, and force behind Jenny Ross Living Foods, including the raw food restaurant 118 Degrees, the popular Raw Basics detox meal programs, and nationwide grocery product line 118 Degrees. She has been an early pioneer of the raw movement, coaching clients about the healing power of living foods, while motivating them to adopt a more vibrant, healthy lifestyle. She has a degree in holistic nutrition and certificates as a health and life coach. Jenny was one of the contributing chefs of *The Daniel Plan Cookbook*.

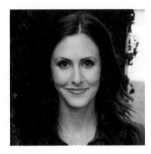

Mareya Ibrahim is best known as "The Fit Foodie." She is an award-winning entrepreneur, television chef, author, and one of The Daniel Plan signature chefs. She is also the CEO and founder of Grow Green Industries, Inc. and cocreator of eatCleaner, the premier lifestyle destination for fit food information. Her book *The Clean Eating Handbook* is touted as the "go-to" guide for anyone looking to eat cleaner and get leaner. She is a featured chef on ABC's Emmy-nominated cooking show *Recipe Rehab,* eHow.com, and Livestrong, and the food expert for San Diego's Channel 6 News.

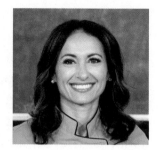

Robert Sturm is one of California's premier chefs and food designers. He has been in the food service industry for more than thirty years, working as an independent consultant to leading restaurant chains around the country. He has been featured in many publications, appears on television and radio, and has been a featured chef at the United Nations, the White House, and the Kremlin. Robert is the three-time winner of the U.S. Chef's Open, a past gold medal member of the U.S. Culinary Olympic Team, and has won many national and international culinary titles and food design awards.

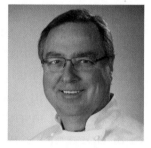

FITNESS TEAM

Tony "The Marine" Lattimore is one of Southern California's premier fitness experts. A skilled personal trainer who privately trains professional athletes, celebrities, and community leaders, he has competed nationally as a bodybuilder. Tony's fitness expertise was featured in P90X and *The Daniel Plan in Action* fitness video series. His powerhouse workouts have a reputation for making fitness fun and exhilarating.

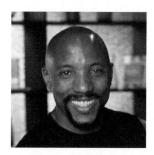

Kevin Forbes has a passion for inspiring others to build healthy habits and push through their physical and mental boundaries. Kevin has helped others grow as a personal trainer, group fitness instructor, and fitness professional. Most recently, he was a featured fitness instructor in *The Daniel Plan in Action* fitness video series. Kevin mentors not only future fitness leaders but also the foster youth in his local community.

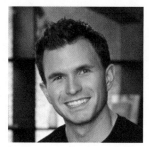

Janet Hertogh shares her love and enthusiasm for teaching in the classroom as an elementary school teacher and in a variety of fitness classes at Saddleback Church. Her passion for life change and transformation is a central theme wherever she goes. Her Masters Degree in Education along with her AFAA and personal training certification make her fully equipped to influence many. Janet was a featured fitness instructor in *The Daniel Plan in Action* fitness video series.

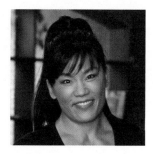

THE ✚ DANIEL PLAN

The Daniel Plan

40 Days to a Healthier Life

*Rick Warren D. Min., Daniel Amen M.D.,
Mark Hyman M.D.*

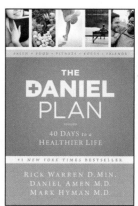

Revolutionize Your Health ... Once and for All.

During an afternoon of baptizing over 800 people, Pastor Rick Warren realized it was time for change. He told his congregation he needed to lose weight and asked if anyone wanted to join him. He thought maybe 200 people would sign up; instead he witnessed a movement unfold as 15,000 people lost over 260,000 pounds in the first year. With assistance from medical and fitness experts, Pastor Rick and thousands of people began a journey to transform their lives.

Welcome to The Daniel Plan.

Here's the secret sauce: The Daniel Plan is designed to be done in a supportive community relying on God's instruction for living.

When it comes to getting healthy, two are always better than one. Our research has revealed that people getting healthy together lose twice as much weight as those who do it alone. God never meant for you to go through life alone and that includes the journey to health.

Unlike the thousands of other books on the market, this book is not about a new diet, guilt-driven gym sessions, or shame-driven fasts. *The Daniel Plan* shows you how the powerful combination of faith, fitness, food, focus, and friends will change your health forever, transforming you in the most head-turning way imaginably—from the inside out.

Available in stores and online!

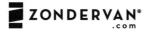

The Daniel Plan Cookbook

Healthy Eating for Life

Rick Warren D. Min., Daniel Amen M.D., and Mark Hyman M.D. featuring The Daniel Plan Signature Chefs

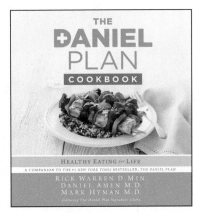

Based on *The Daniel Plan* book, *The Daniel Plan Cookbook: 40 Days to a Healthier Life* is a beautiful four-color cookbook filled with more than 100 delicious, Daniel Plan-approved recipes that offer an abundance of options to bring healthy cooking into your kitchen.

No boring drinks or bland entrées here. Get ready to enjoy appetizing, inviting, clean, simple meals to share in community with your friends and family.

Healthy cooking can be easy and delicious, and *The Daniel Plan Cookbook* is the mouth-watering companion to *The Daniel Plan* book and *The Daniel Plan Journal* to help transform your health in the most head-turning way imaginably—from the inside out.

Available in stores and online!

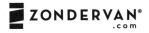

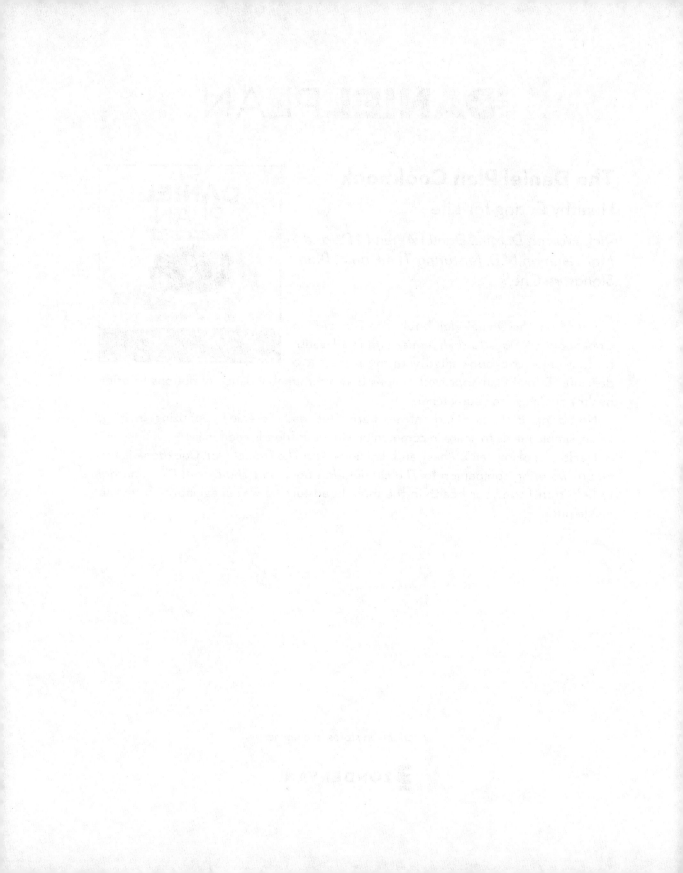

THE +DANIELPLAN

The Daniel Plan Journal

40 Days to a Healthier Life

Rick Warren and The Daniel Plan Team

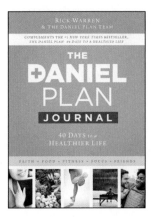

The Perfect Daniel Plan Companion for Better Overall Health

Research shows that tracking your food and exercise greatly contributes to your long-term success. Maximize your momentum by exploring and charting your journey through the five key Essentials of The Daniel Plan — Faith, Food, Fitness, Focus, and Friends.

Taking readers of *The Daniel Plan: 40 Days to a Healthier Life* to the next level, *The Daniel Plan Journal* is the perfect companion, providing encouraging reminders about your health. On the days you need a little boost, *The Daniel Plan Journal* has the daily Scripture, inspiration, and motivation you need to stay on track and keep moving forward.

Available in stores and online!

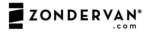
ZONDERVAN®
.com

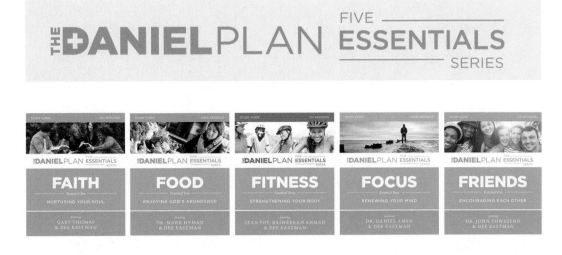

The Daniel Plan Five Essentials Series

The Daniel Plan Five Essentials Series is an innovative approach to creating a healthy lifestyle, rooted and framed by five life areas: Faith, Food, Fitness, Focus, and Friends.

Host Dee Eastman and The Daniel Plan's founding doctors and wellness faculty — including Gary Thomas, Dr. Mark Hyman, Sean Foy, Basheerah Ahmad, Dr. Daniel Amen, and Dr. John Townsend — equip you to make healthy choices on a daily basis.

Each video session features not only great teaching but testimony from those who have incorporated The Daniel Plan into their everyday lives. A weekly Fitness Move and Food Tip are also provided. The study guide include icebreakers and review questions, video notes, video discussion questions, next steps suggestions, prayer starters, and helpful appendices.

The Daniel Plan has transformed thousands of people around the world and it can transform you as well.

Available in stores and online!

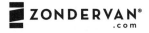

The Daniel Plan in Action

40 Day Fitness Programs With Dynamic Workouts

Introduction by Rick Warren D. Min.

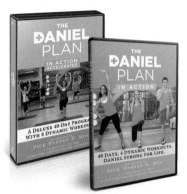

The Daniel Plan in Action is a 40-day fitness system with an innovative approach to creating a healthy lifestyle, rooted and framed by five life areas: faith, food, fitness, focus and friends. Three expert instructors lead the variety of inspiring workouts with a strong backbone of faith and community, complemented by a soundtrack of exclusive Christian music. This 4-session and 8-session systems focus on an abundance of healthy choices offering you the encouragement and inspiration you need to succeed.

Go to DanielPlan.com now to learn more.

The Daniel Plan Jumpstart Guide

Daily Steps to a Healthier Life

Rick Warren D. Min., Daniel Amen M.D., Mark Hyman M.D.

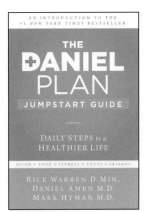

The Daniel Plan Jumpstart Guide provides a bird's-eye view of getting your life on track to better health in five key areas: Faith, Food, Fitness, Focus, and Friends. This booklet provides all the key principles for readers to gain a vision for health and get started—breaking out existing content from *The Daniel Plan: 40 Days to a Healthier Life* into a 40-day action plan. The *Jumpstart Guide* encourages readers to use *The Daniel Plan* and *The Daniel Plan Journal* for more information and further success.

Available in stores and online!

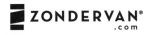